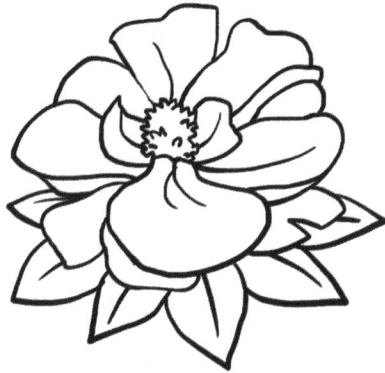

I0146483

PROPERTY OF

_____

_____

_____

DEDICATION

This Massage Therapist Appointment Book is dedicated to all the massage therapists out there who want to record all their clients appointments and document their findings in the process.

You are my inspiration for producing books and I'm honored to be a part of keeping all of your client notes and records organized.

This journal notebook will help you record the details of your massage therapy business.

Thoughtfully put together with these sections to record: Name, Date, Time, Phone, E-mail, Service, Supplies, Duration, Notes, & Body Diagram.

HOW TO USE THIS BOOK

The purpose of this book is to keep all of your Massage Therapist notes all in one place. It will help keep you organized.

This Massage Therapist Appointment Book will allow you to accurately document every detail about client appointments.

Here are examples of the prompts for you to fill in and write about your experience in this book:

1. Client Name
2. Date
3. Time
4. Phone
5. E-mail
6. Service
7. Supplies
8. Duration
9. Notes
10. Body Diagram With Notes

CLIENT

DATE	TIME
PHONE	EMAIL
SERVICE	DURATION

SUPPLIES

NOTES

CLIENT

DATE	TIME
PHONE	EMAIL
SERVICE	DURATION

SUPPLIES

NOTES

CLIENT

DATE	TIME
PHONE	EMAIL
SERVICE	DURATION

SUPPLIES

NOTES

CLIENT

DATE	TIME
PHONE	EMAIL
SERVICE	DURATION

SUPPLIES

NOTES

CLIENT

DATE	TIME
PHONE	EMAIL
SERVICE	DURATION

SUPPLIES

NOTES

CLIENT

DATE	TIME
PHONE	EMAIL
SERVICE	DURATION

SUPPLIES

NOTES

CLIENT

DATE	TIME
PHONE	EMAIL
SERVICE	DURATION

SUPPLIES

NOTES

CLIENT

DATE	TIME
PHONE	EMAIL
SERVICE	DURATION

SUPPLIES

NOTES

CLIENT

DATE	TIME
PHONE	EMAIL
SERVICE	DURATION

SUPPLIES

NOTES

CLIENT

DATE	TIME
PHONE	EMAIL
SERVICE	DURATION

SUPPLIES

NOTES

CLIENT

DATE	TIME
PHONE	EMAIL
SERVICE	DURATION

SUPPLIES

NOTES

CLIENT

DATE	TIME
PHONE	EMAIL
SERVICE	DURATION

SUPPLIES

NOTES

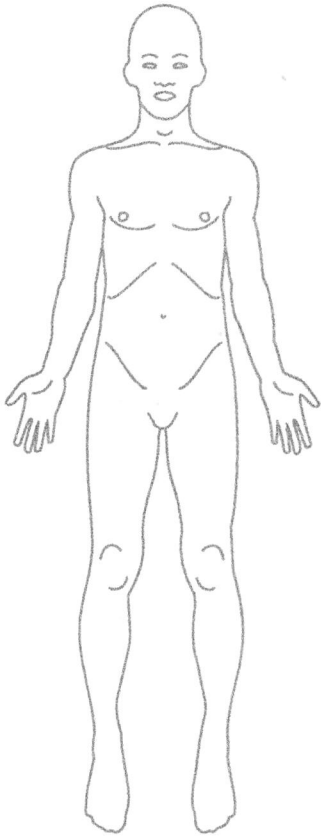

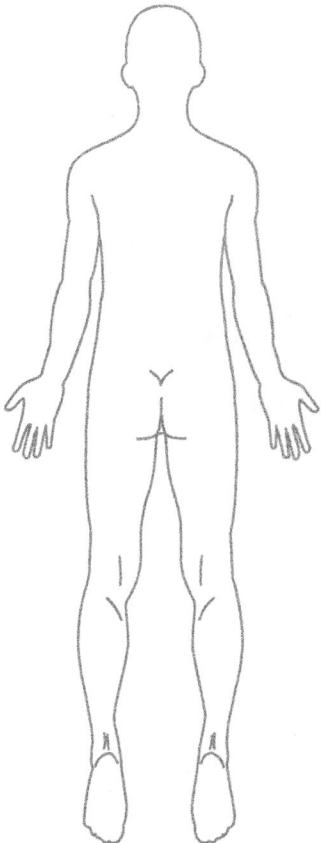

CLIENT

DATE	TIME
PHONE	EMAIL
SERVICE	DURATION

SUPPLIES

NOTES

CLIENT

DATE	TIME
PHONE	EMAIL
SERVICE	DURATION

SUPPLIES

NOTES

CLIENT

DATE	TIME
PHONE	EMAIL
SERVICE	DURATION

SUPPLIES

NOTES

CLIENT

DATE	TIME
PHONE	EMAIL
SERVICE	DURATION

SUPPLIES

NOTES

CLIENT

DATE	TIME
PHONE	EMAIL
SERVICE	DURATION

SUPPLIES

NOTES

CLIENT

DATE	TIME
PHONE	EMAIL
SERVICE	DURATION

SUPPLIES

NOTES

CLIENT

DATE	TIME
PHONE	EMAIL
SERVICE	DURATION

SUPPLIES

NOTES

CLIENT

DATE	TIME
PHONE	EMAIL
SERVICE	DURATION

SUPPLIES

NOTES

CLIENT

DATE	TIME
PHONE	EMAIL
SERVICE	DURATION

SUPPLIES

NOTES

CLIENT

DATE	TIME
PHONE	EMAIL
SERVICE	DURATION

SUPPLIES

NOTES

CLIENT

DATE	TIME
PHONE	EMAIL
SERVICE	DURATION

SUPPLIES

NOTES

CLIENT

DATE	TIME
PHONE	EMAIL
SERVICE	DURATION

SUPPLIES

NOTES

CLIENT

DATE | TIME

PHONE | EMAIL

SERVICE | DURATION

SUPPLIES

NOTES

CLIENT

DATE | TIME

PHONE | EMAIL

SERVICE | DURATION

SUPPLIES

NOTES

CLIENT

DATE | TIME

PHONE | EMAIL

SERVICE | DURATION

SUPPLIES

NOTES

CLIENT

DATE | TIME

PHONE | EMAIL

SERVICE | DURATION

SUPPLIES

NOTES

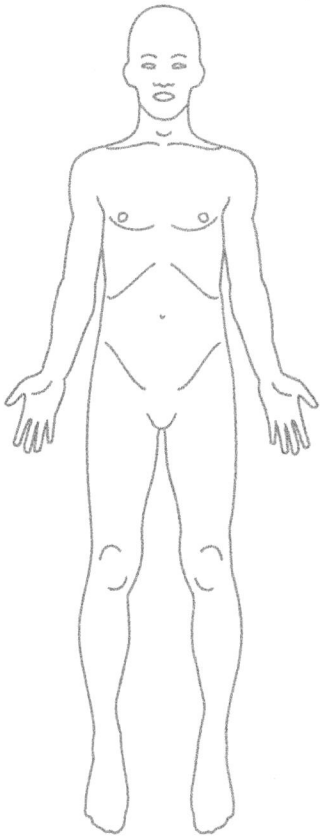

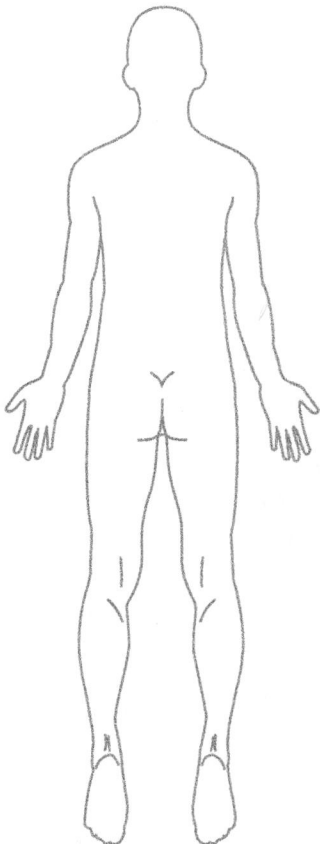

NOTES

_____

_____

_____

_____

_____

_____

_____

_____

_____

_____

_____

_____

_____

_____

_____

_____

_____

_____

_____

_____

_____

_____

_____

_____

_____

_____

_____

CLIENT

DATE	TIME
PHONE	EMAIL
SERVICE	DURATION

SUPPLIES

NOTES

CLIENT

DATE	TIME
PHONE	EMAIL
SERVICE	DURATION

SUPPLIES

NOTES

CLIENT

DATE	TIME
PHONE	EMAIL
SERVICE	DURATION

SUPPLIES

NOTES

CLIENT

DATE	TIME
PHONE	EMAIL
SERVICE	DURATION

SUPPLIES

NOTES

CLIENT

DATE	TIME
PHONE	EMAIL
SERVICE	DURATION

SUPPLIES

NOTES

CLIENT

DATE	TIME
PHONE	EMAIL
SERVICE	DURATION

SUPPLIES

NOTES

CLIENT

DATE	TIME
PHONE	EMAIL
SERVICE	DURATION

SUPPLIES

NOTES

CLIENT

DATE	TIME
PHONE	EMAIL
SERVICE	DURATION

SUPPLIES

NOTES

CLIENT

DATE	TIME
PHONE	EMAIL
SERVICE	DURATION

SUPPLIES

NOTES

CLIENT

DATE	TIME
PHONE	EMAIL
SERVICE	DURATION

SUPPLIES

NOTES

CLIENT

DATE	TIME
PHONE	EMAIL
SERVICE	DURATION

SUPPLIES

NOTES

CLIENT

DATE	TIME
PHONE	EMAIL
SERVICE	DURATION

SUPPLIES

NOTES

CLIENT

DATE	TIME
PHONE	EMAIL
SERVICE	DURATION

SUPPLIES

NOTES

CLIENT

DATE	TIME
PHONE	EMAIL
SERVICE	DURATION

SUPPLIES

NOTES

CLIENT

DATE	TIME
PHONE	EMAIL
SERVICE	DURATION

SUPPLIES

NOTES

CLIENT

DATE	TIME
PHONE	EMAIL
SERVICE	DURATION

SUPPLIES

NOTES

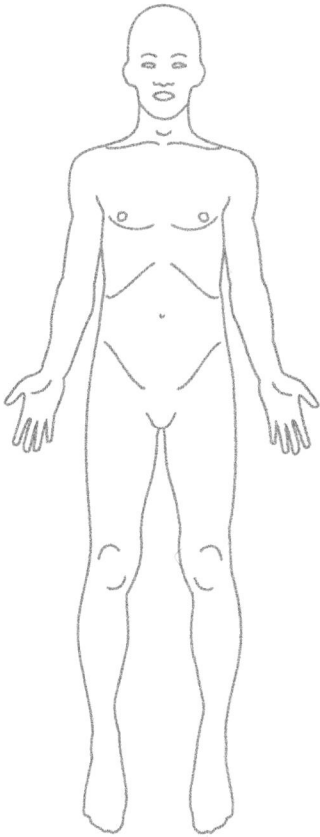

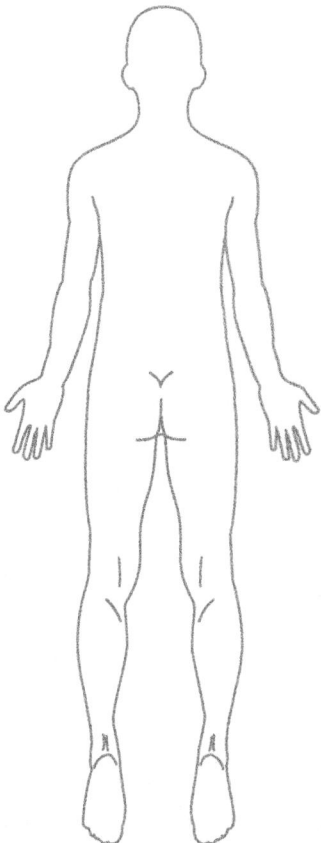

NOTES

CLIENT

DATE	TIME
PHONE	EMAIL
SERVICE	DURATION

SUPPLIES

NOTES

CLIENT

DATE	TIME
PHONE	EMAIL
SERVICE	DURATION

SUPPLIES

NOTES

CLIENT

DATE	TIME
PHONE	EMAIL
SERVICE	DURATION

SUPPLIES

NOTES

CLIENT

DATE	TIME
PHONE	EMAIL
SERVICE	DURATION

SUPPLIES

NOTES

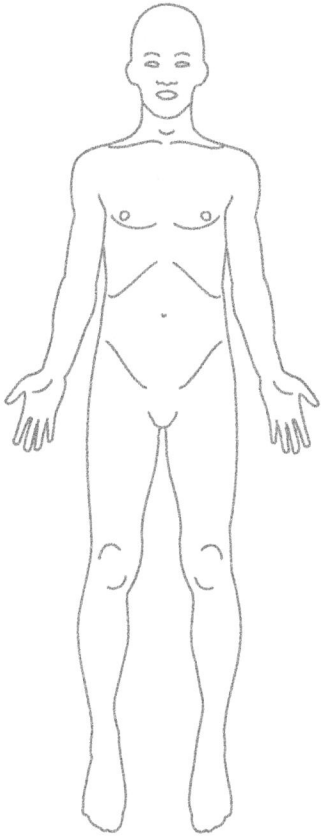

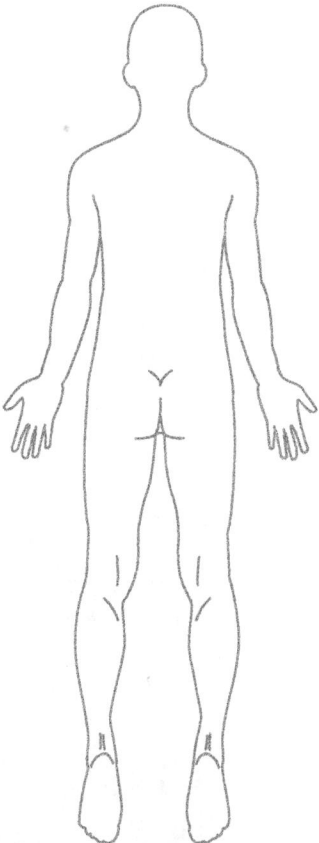

CLIENT

DATE	TIME
PHONE	EMAIL
SERVICE	DURATION

SUPPLIES

NOTES

CLIENT

DATE	TIME
PHONE	EMAIL
SERVICE	DURATION

SUPPLIES

NOTES

CLIENT

DATE	TIME
PHONE	EMAIL
SERVICE	DURATION

SUPPLIES

NOTES

CLIENT

DATE	TIME
PHONE	EMAIL
SERVICE	DURATION

SUPPLIES

NOTES

CLIENT

DATE	TIME
PHONE	EMAIL
SERVICE	DURATION

SUPPLIES

NOTES

CLIENT

DATE	TIME
PHONE	EMAIL
SERVICE	DURATION

SUPPLIES

NOTES

CLIENT

DATE	TIME
PHONE	EMAIL
SERVICE	DURATION

SUPPLIES

NOTES

CLIENT

DATE	TIME
PHONE	EMAIL
SERVICE	DURATION

SUPPLIES

NOTES

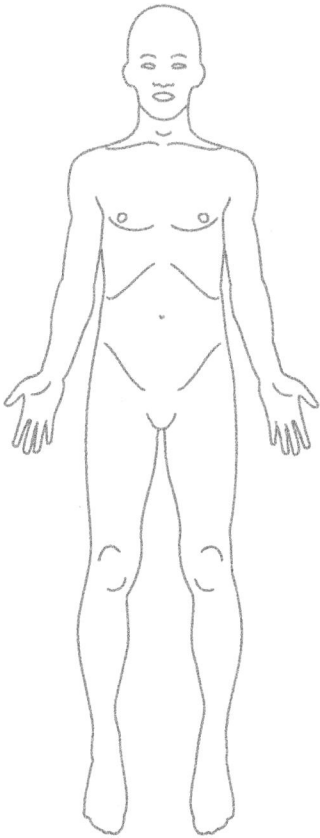

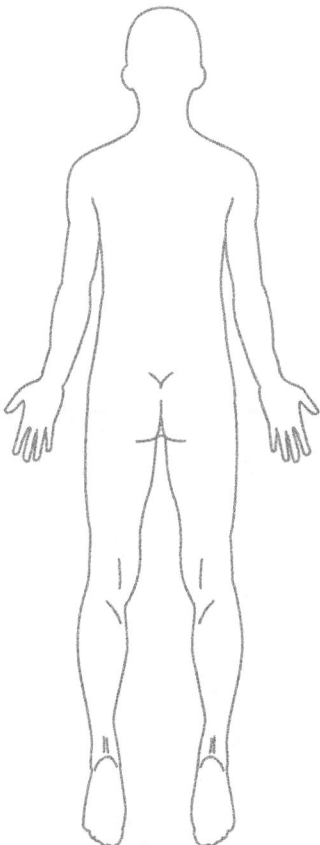

CLIENT

DATE	TIME
PHONE	EMAIL
SERVICE	DURATION

SUPPLIES

NOTES

CLIENT

DATE	TIME
PHONE	EMAIL
SERVICE	DURATION

SUPPLIES

NOTES

CLIENT

DATE	TIME
PHONE	EMAIL
SERVICE	DURATION

SUPPLIES

NOTES

CLIENT

DATE	TIME
PHONE	EMAIL
SERVICE	DURATION

SUPPLIES

NOTES

NOTES

CLIENT

DATE	TIME
PHONE	EMAIL
SERVICE	DURATION

SUPPLIES

NOTES

CLIENT

DATE	TIME
PHONE	EMAIL
SERVICE	DURATION

SUPPLIES

NOTES

CLIENT

DATE	TIME
PHONE	EMAIL
SERVICE	DURATION

SUPPLIES

NOTES

CLIENT

DATE	TIME
PHONE	EMAIL
SERVICE	DURATION

SUPPLIES

NOTES

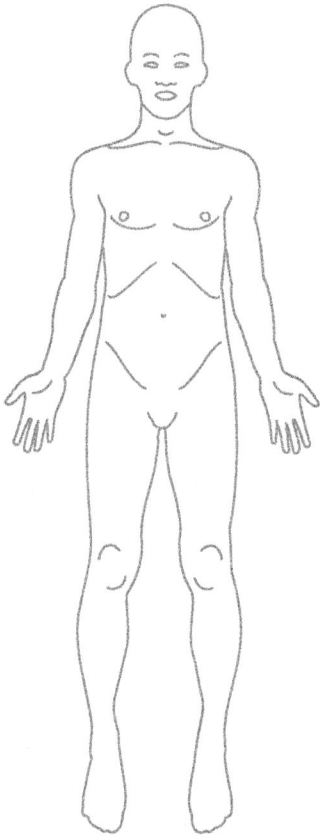

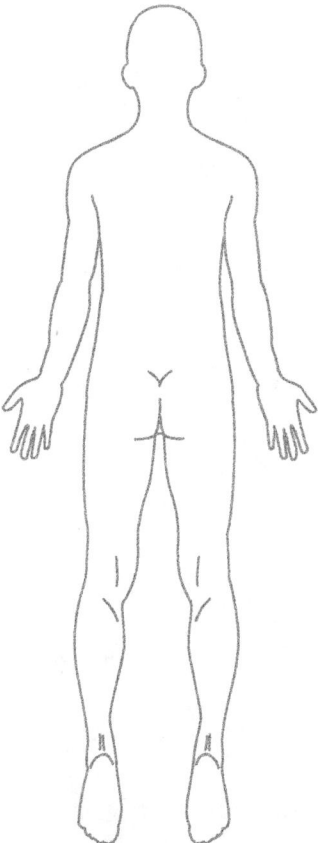

CLIENT

DATE | TIME

PHONE | EMAIL

SERVICE | DURATION

SUPPLIES

NOTES

CLIENT

DATE | TIME

PHONE | EMAIL

SERVICE | DURATION

SUPPLIES

NOTES

CLIENT

DATE | TIME

PHONE | EMAIL

SERVICE | DURATION

SUPPLIES

NOTES

CLIENT

DATE | TIME

PHONE | EMAIL

SERVICE | DURATION

SUPPLIES

NOTES

CLIENT

DATE	TIME
PHONE	EMAIL
SERVICE	DURATION

SUPPLIES

NOTES

CLIENT

DATE	TIME
PHONE	EMAIL
SERVICE	DURATION

SUPPLIES

NOTES

CLIENT

DATE	TIME
PHONE	EMAIL
SERVICE	DURATION

SUPPLIES

NOTES

CLIENT

DATE	TIME
PHONE	EMAIL
SERVICE	DURATION

SUPPLIES

NOTES

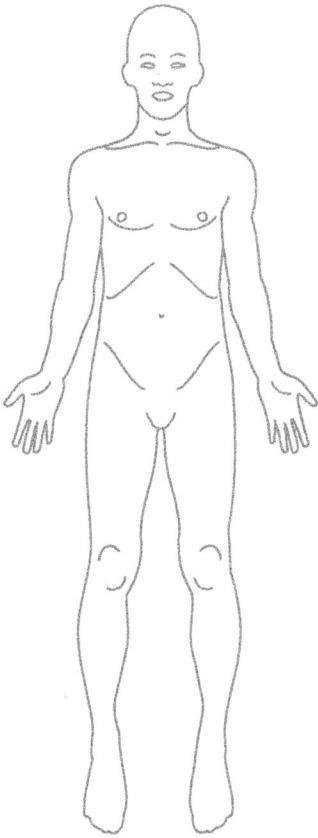

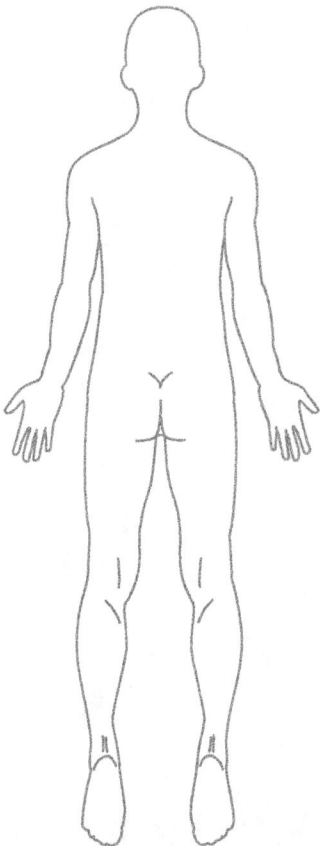

NOTES

_____

_____

_____

_____

_____

_____

_____

_____

_____

_____

_____

_____

_____

_____

_____

_____

_____

_____

_____

_____

_____

_____

_____

_____

_____

_____

_____

_____

CLIENT

DATE	TIME
PHONE	EMAIL
SERVICE	DURATION

SUPPLIES

NOTES

CLIENT

DATE	TIME
PHONE	EMAIL
SERVICE	DURATION

SUPPLIES

NOTES

CLIENT

DATE	TIME
PHONE	EMAIL
SERVICE	DURATION

SUPPLIES

NOTES

CLIENT

DATE	TIME
PHONE	EMAIL
SERVICE	DURATION

SUPPLIES

NOTES

CLIENT

DATE	TIME
PHONE	EMAIL
SERVICE	DURATION

SUPPLIES

NOTES

CLIENT

DATE	TIME
PHONE	EMAIL
SERVICE	DURATION

SUPPLIES

NOTES

CLIENT

DATE	TIME
PHONE	EMAIL
SERVICE	DURATION

SUPPLIES

NOTES

CLIENT

DATE	TIME
PHONE	EMAIL
SERVICE	DURATION

SUPPLIES

NOTES

CLIENT

DATE	TIME
PHONE	EMAIL
SERVICE	DURATION

SUPPLIES

NOTES

CLIENT

DATE	TIME
PHONE	EMAIL
SERVICE	DURATION

SUPPLIES

NOTES

CLIENT

DATE	TIME
PHONE	EMAIL
SERVICE	DURATION

SUPPLIES

NOTES

CLIENT

DATE	TIME
PHONE	EMAIL
SERVICE	DURATION

SUPPLIES

NOTES

CLIENT

DATE	TIME
PHONE	EMAIL
SERVICE	DURATION

SUPPLIES

NOTES

CLIENT

DATE	TIME
PHONE	EMAIL
SERVICE	DURATION

SUPPLIES

NOTES

CLIENT

DATE	TIME
PHONE	EMAIL
SERVICE	DURATION

SUPPLIES

NOTES

CLIENT

DATE	TIME
PHONE	EMAIL
SERVICE	DURATION

SUPPLIES

NOTES

CLIENT

DATE	TIME
PHONE	EMAIL
SERVICE	DURATION

SUPPLIES

NOTES

CLIENT

DATE	TIME
PHONE	EMAIL
SERVICE	DURATION

SUPPLIES

NOTES

CLIENT

DATE	TIME
PHONE	EMAIL
SERVICE	DURATION

SUPPLIES

NOTES

CLIENT

DATE	TIME
PHONE	EMAIL
SERVICE	DURATION

SUPPLIES

NOTES

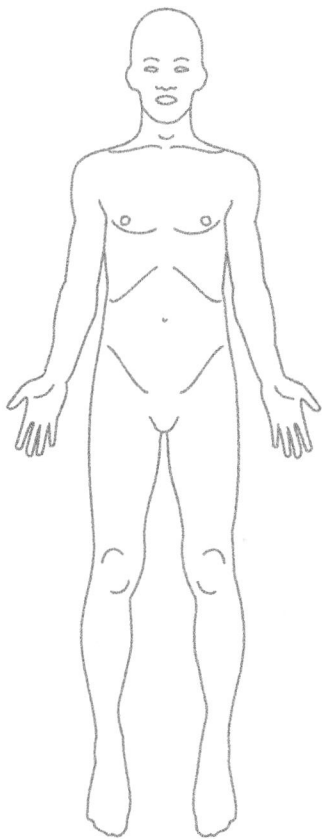

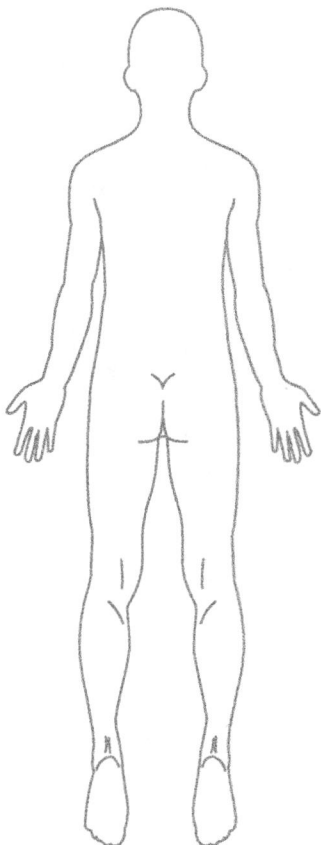

CLIENT

DATE	TIME
PHONE	EMAIL
SERVICE	DURATION

SUPPLIES

NOTES

CLIENT

DATE	TIME
PHONE	EMAIL
SERVICE	DURATION

SUPPLIES

NOTES

CLIENT

DATE	TIME
PHONE	EMAIL
SERVICE	DURATION

SUPPLIES

NOTES

CLIENT

DATE	TIME
PHONE	EMAIL
SERVICE	DURATION

SUPPLIES

NOTES

CLIENT

DATE	TIME
PHONE	EMAIL
SERVICE	DURATION

SUPPLIES

NOTES

CLIENT

DATE	TIME
PHONE	EMAIL
SERVICE	DURATION

SUPPLIES

NOTES

CLIENT

DATE	TIME
PHONE	EMAIL
SERVICE	DURATION

SUPPLIES

NOTES

CLIENT

DATE	TIME
PHONE	EMAIL
SERVICE	DURATION

SUPPLIES

NOTES

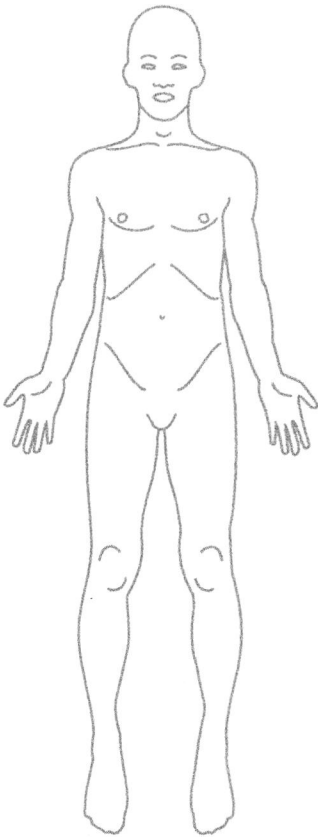

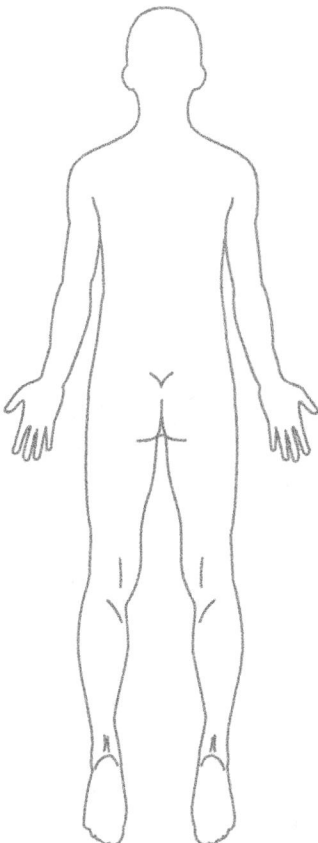

NOTES

CLIENT

DATE	TIME
PHONE	EMAIL
SERVICE	DURATION

SUPPLIES

NOTES

CLIENT

DATE	TIME
PHONE	EMAIL
SERVICE	DURATION

SUPPLIES

NOTES

CLIENT

DATE	TIME
PHONE	EMAIL
SERVICE	DURATION

SUPPLIES

NOTES

CLIENT

DATE	TIME
PHONE	EMAIL
SERVICE	DURATION

SUPPLIES

NOTES

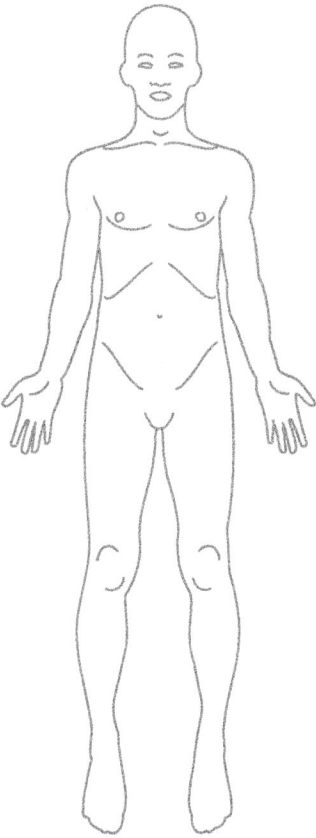

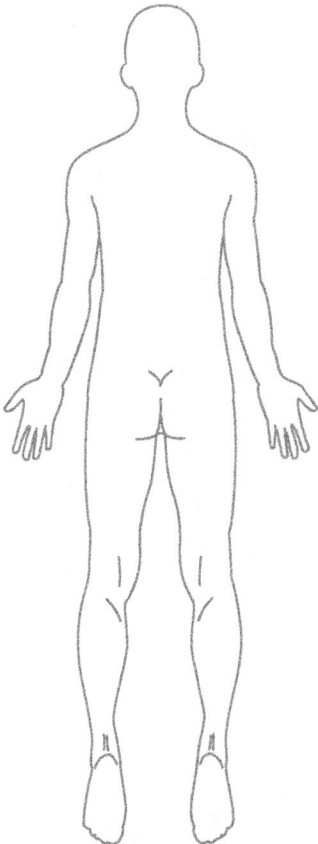

CLIENT

DATE	TIME
PHONE	EMAIL
SERVICE	DURATION

SUPPLIES

NOTES

CLIENT

DATE	TIME
PHONE	EMAIL
SERVICE	DURATION

SUPPLIES

NOTES

CLIENT

DATE	TIME
PHONE	EMAIL
SERVICE	DURATION

SUPPLIES

NOTES

CLIENT

DATE	TIME
PHONE	EMAIL
SERVICE	DURATION

SUPPLIES

NOTES

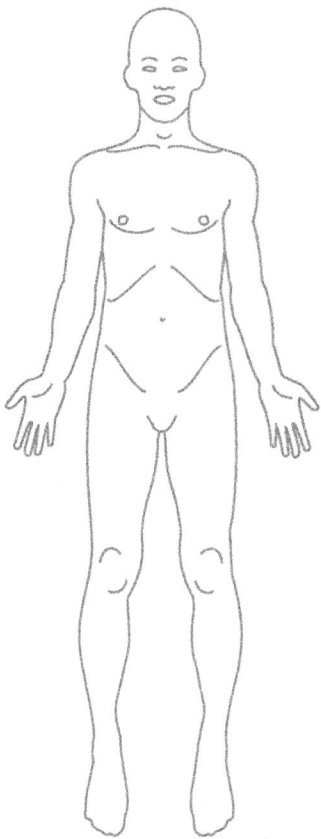

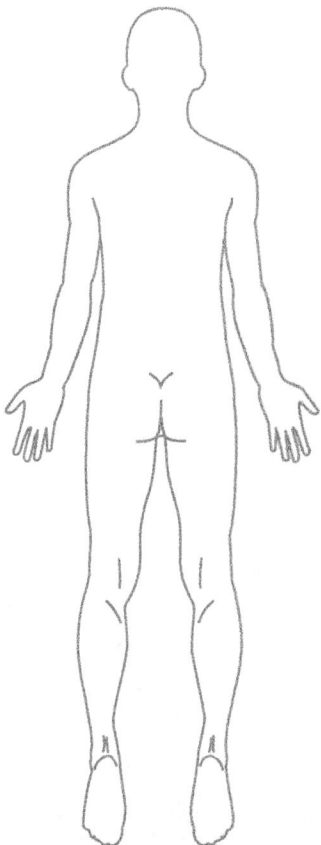

NOTES

_____

_____

_____

_____

_____

_____

_____

_____

_____

_____

_____

_____

_____

_____

_____

_____

_____

_____

_____

_____

_____

_____

_____

_____

CLIENT

DATE	TIME
PHONE	EMAIL
SERVICE	DURATION

SUPPLIES

NOTES

CLIENT

DATE	TIME
PHONE	EMAIL
SERVICE	DURATION

SUPPLIES

NOTES

CLIENT

DATE	TIME
PHONE	EMAIL
SERVICE	DURATION

SUPPLIES

NOTES

CLIENT

DATE	TIME
PHONE	EMAIL
SERVICE	DURATION

SUPPLIES

NOTES

CLIENT

DATE | TIME

PHONE | EMAIL

SERVICE | DURATION

SUPPLIES

NOTES

CLIENT

DATE | TIME

PHONE | EMAIL

SERVICE | DURATION

SUPPLIES

NOTES

CLIENT

DATE | TIME

PHONE | EMAIL

SERVICE | DURATION

SUPPLIES

NOTES

CLIENT

DATE | TIME

PHONE | EMAIL

SERVICE | DURATION

SUPPLIES

NOTES

CLIENT

DATE	TIME
PHONE	EMAIL
SERVICE	DURATION

SUPPLIES

NOTES

CLIENT

DATE	TIME
PHONE	EMAIL
SERVICE	DURATION

SUPPLIES

NOTES

CLIENT

DATE	TIME
PHONE	EMAIL
SERVICE	DURATION

SUPPLIES

NOTES

CLIENT

DATE	TIME
PHONE	EMAIL
SERVICE	DURATION

SUPPLIES

NOTES

CLIENT

DATE	TIME
PHONE	EMAIL
SERVICE	DURATION

SUPPLIES

NOTES

CLIENT

DATE	TIME
PHONE	EMAIL
SERVICE	DURATION

SUPPLIES

NOTES

CLIENT

DATE	TIME
PHONE	EMAIL
SERVICE	DURATION

SUPPLIES

NOTES

CLIENT

DATE	TIME
PHONE	EMAIL
SERVICE	DURATION

SUPPLIES

NOTES

CLIENT

DATE	TIME
PHONE	EMAIL
SERVICE	DURATION

SUPPLIES

NOTES

CLIENT

DATE	TIME
PHONE	EMAIL
SERVICE	DURATION

SUPPLIES

NOTES

CLIENT

DATE	TIME
PHONE	EMAIL
SERVICE	DURATION

SUPPLIES

NOTES

CLIENT

DATE	TIME
PHONE	EMAIL
SERVICE	DURATION

SUPPLIES

NOTES

CLIENT

DATE | TIME

PHONE | EMAIL

SERVICE | DURATION

SUPPLIES

NOTES

CLIENT

DATE | TIME

PHONE | EMAIL

SERVICE | DURATION

SUPPLIES

NOTES

CLIENT

DATE | TIME

PHONE | EMAIL

SERVICE | DURATION

SUPPLIES

NOTES

CLIENT

DATE | TIME

PHONE | EMAIL

SERVICE | DURATION

SUPPLIES

NOTES

CLIENT

DATE

TIME

PHONE

EMAIL

SERVICE

DURATION

SUPPLIES

NOTES

CLIENT

DATE

TIME

PHONE

EMAIL

SERVICE

DURATION

SUPPLIES

NOTES

CLIENT

DATE

TIME

PHONE

EMAIL

SERVICE

DURATION

SUPPLIES

NOTES

CLIENT

DATE

TIME

PHONE

EMAIL

SERVICE

DURATION

SUPPLIES

NOTES

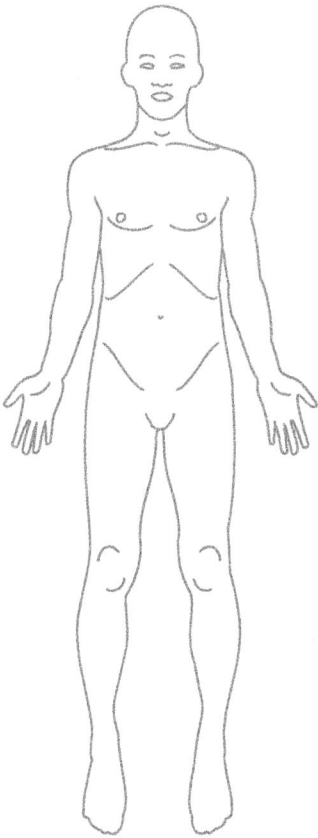

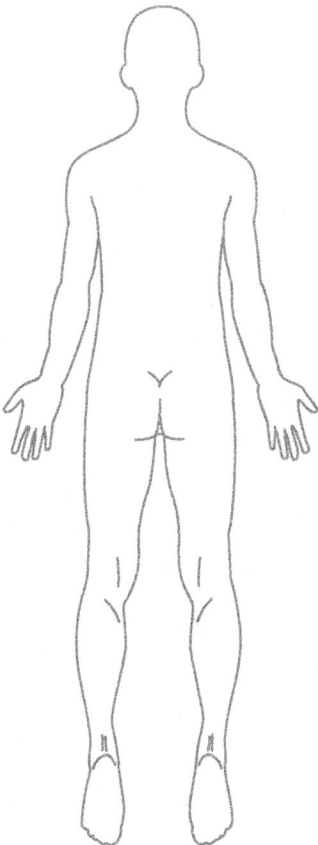

NOTES

CLIENT

DATE	TIME
PHONE	EMAIL
SERVICE	DURATION

SUPPLIES

NOTES

CLIENT

DATE	TIME
PHONE	EMAIL
SERVICE	DURATION

SUPPLIES

NOTES

CLIENT

DATE	TIME
PHONE	EMAIL
SERVICE	DURATION

SUPPLIES

NOTES

CLIENT

DATE	TIME
PHONE	EMAIL
SERVICE	DURATION

SUPPLIES

NOTES

CLIENT

DATE	TIME
PHONE	EMAIL
SERVICE	DURATION

SUPPLIES

NOTES

CLIENT

DATE	TIME
PHONE	EMAIL
SERVICE	DURATION

SUPPLIES

NOTES

CLIENT

DATE	TIME
PHONE	EMAIL
SERVICE	DURATION

SUPPLIES

NOTES

CLIENT

DATE	TIME
PHONE	EMAIL
SERVICE	DURATION

SUPPLIES

NOTES

CLIENT

DATE	TIME
PHONE	EMAIL
SERVICE	DURATION

SUPPLIES

NOTES

CLIENT

DATE	TIME
PHONE	EMAIL
SERVICE	DURATION

SUPPLIES

NOTES

CLIENT

DATE	TIME
PHONE	EMAIL
SERVICE	DURATION

SUPPLIES

NOTES

CLIENT

DATE	TIME
PHONE	EMAIL
SERVICE	DURATION

SUPPLIES

NOTES

CLIENT

DATE | TIME

PHONE | EMAIL

SERVICE | DURATION

SUPPLIES

NOTES

CLIENT

DATE | TIME

PHONE | EMAIL

SERVICE | DURATION

SUPPLIES

NOTES

CLIENT

DATE | TIME

PHONE | EMAIL

SERVICE | DURATION

SUPPLIES

NOTES

CLIENT

DATE | TIME

PHONE | EMAIL

SERVICE | DURATION

SUPPLIES

NOTES

CLIENT

DATE	TIME
PHONE	EMAIL
SERVICE	DURATION

SUPPLIES

NOTES

CLIENT

DATE	TIME
PHONE	EMAIL
SERVICE	DURATION

SUPPLIES

NOTES

CLIENT

DATE	TIME
PHONE	EMAIL
SERVICE	DURATION

SUPPLIES

NOTES

CLIENT

DATE	TIME
PHONE	EMAIL
SERVICE	DURATION

SUPPLIES

NOTES

CLIENT

DATE	TIME
PHONE	EMAIL
SERVICE	DURATION

SUPPLIES

NOTES

CLIENT

DATE	TIME
PHONE	EMAIL
SERVICE	DURATION

SUPPLIES

NOTES

CLIENT

DATE	TIME
PHONE	EMAIL
SERVICE	DURATION

SUPPLIES

NOTES

CLIENT

DATE	TIME
PHONE	EMAIL
SERVICE	DURATION

SUPPLIES

NOTES

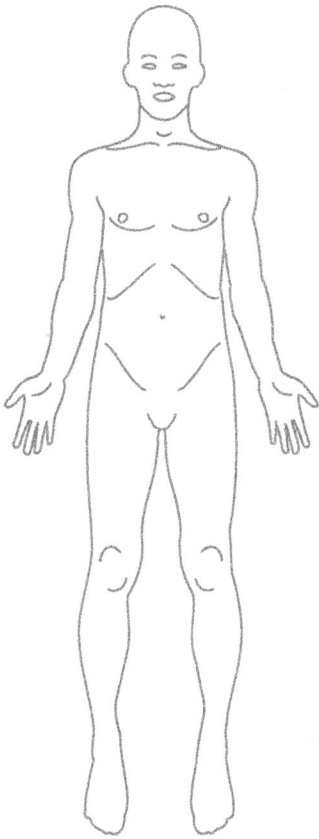

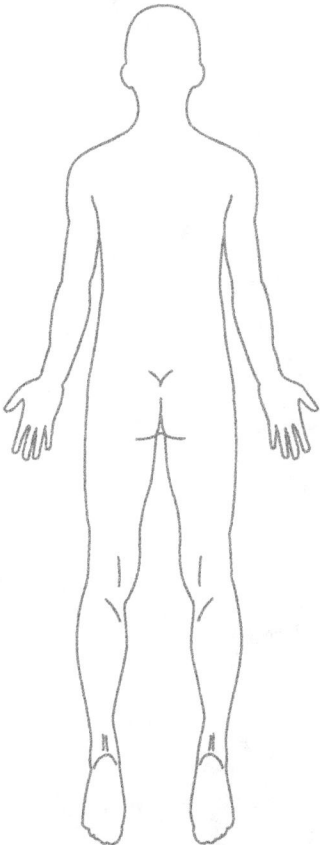

NOTES

_____
_____
_____
_____
_____
_____
_____
_____
_____
_____
_____
_____
_____
_____
_____
_____
_____
_____
_____
_____
_____
_____
_____
_____
_____
_____
_____

CLIENT

DATE	TIME
PHONE	EMAIL
SERVICE	DURATION

SUPPLIES

NOTES

CLIENT

DATE	TIME
PHONE	EMAIL
SERVICE	DURATION

SUPPLIES

NOTES

CLIENT

DATE	TIME
PHONE	EMAIL
SERVICE	DURATION

SUPPLIES

NOTES

CLIENT

DATE	TIME
PHONE	EMAIL
SERVICE	DURATION

SUPPLIES

NOTES

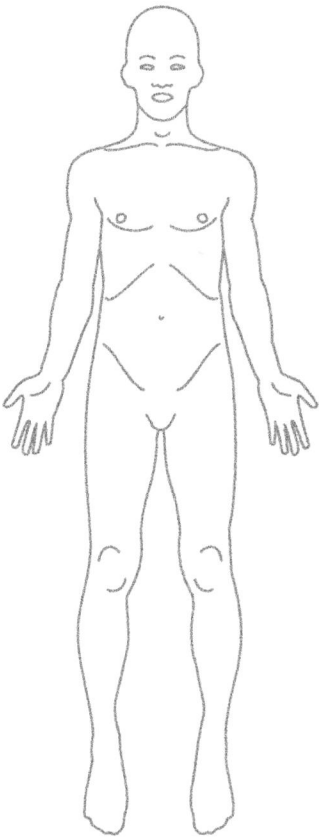

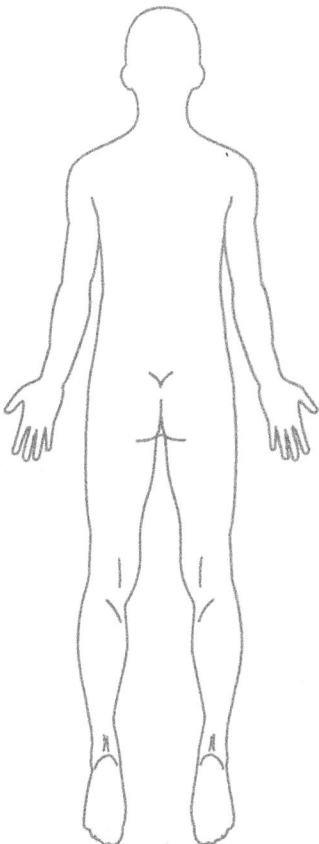

NOTES

CLIENT

DATE	TIME
PHONE	EMAIL
SERVICE	DURATION

SUPPLIES

NOTES

CLIENT

DATE	TIME
PHONE	EMAIL
SERVICE	DURATION

SUPPLIES

NOTES

CLIENT

DATE	TIME
PHONE	EMAIL
SERVICE	DURATION

SUPPLIES

NOTES

CLIENT

DATE	TIME
PHONE	EMAIL
SERVICE	DURATION

SUPPLIES

NOTES

CLIENT

DATE	TIME
PHONE	EMAIL
SERVICE	DURATION

SUPPLIES

NOTES

CLIENT

DATE	TIME
PHONE	EMAIL
SERVICE	DURATION

SUPPLIES

NOTES

CLIENT

DATE	TIME
PHONE	EMAIL
SERVICE	DURATION

SUPPLIES

NOTES

CLIENT

DATE	TIME
PHONE	EMAIL
SERVICE	DURATION

SUPPLIES

NOTES

CLIENT

DATE	TIME
PHONE	EMAIL
SERVICE	DURATION

SUPPLIES

NOTES

CLIENT

DATE	TIME
PHONE	EMAIL
SERVICE	DURATION

SUPPLIES

NOTES

CLIENT

DATE	TIME
PHONE	EMAIL
SERVICE	DURATION

SUPPLIES

NOTES

CLIENT

DATE	TIME
PHONE	EMAIL
SERVICE	DURATION

SUPPLIES

NOTES

CLIENT

DATE	TIME
PHONE	EMAIL
SERVICE	DURATION

SUPPLIES

NOTES

CLIENT

DATE	TIME
PHONE	EMAIL
SERVICE	DURATION

SUPPLIES

NOTES

CLIENT

DATE	TIME
PHONE	EMAIL
SERVICE	DURATION

SUPPLIES

NOTES

CLIENT

DATE	TIME
PHONE	EMAIL
SERVICE	DURATION

SUPPLIES

NOTES

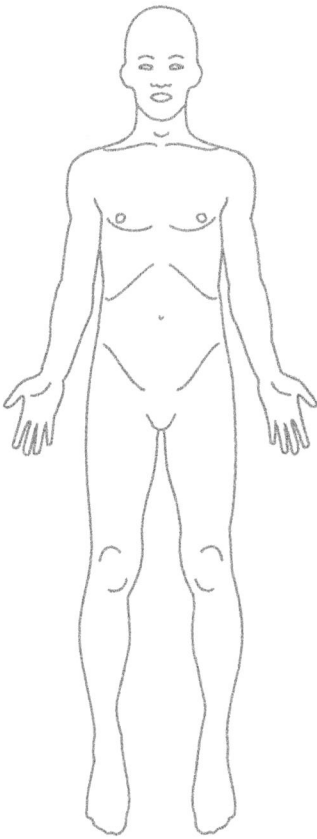

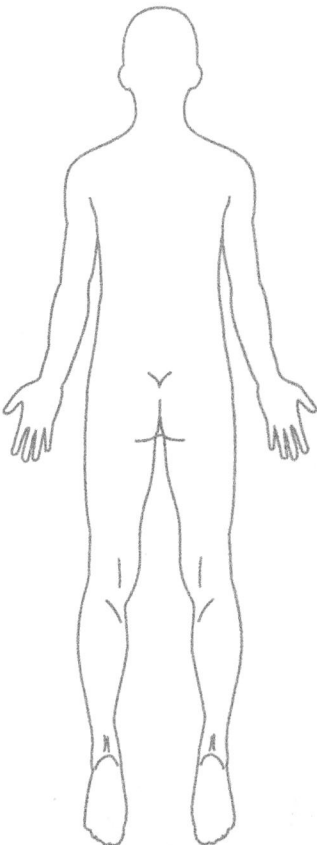

CLIENT

DATE	TIME
PHONE	EMAIL
SERVICE	DURATION

SUPPLIES

NOTES

CLIENT

DATE	TIME
PHONE	EMAIL
SERVICE	DURATION

SUPPLIES

NOTES

CLIENT

DATE	TIME
PHONE	EMAIL
SERVICE	DURATION

SUPPLIES

NOTES

CLIENT

DATE	TIME
PHONE	EMAIL
SERVICE	DURATION

SUPPLIES

NOTES

CLIENT

DATE | TIME

PHONE | EMAIL

SERVICE | DURATION

SUPPLIES

NOTES

CLIENT

DATE | TIME

PHONE | EMAIL

SERVICE | DURATION

SUPPLIES

NOTES

CLIENT

DATE | TIME

PHONE | EMAIL

SERVICE | DURATION

SUPPLIES

NOTES

CLIENT

DATE | TIME

PHONE | EMAIL

SERVICE | DURATION

SUPPLIES

NOTES

CLIENT

DATE | TIME

PHONE | EMAIL

SERVICE | DURATION

SUPPLIES

NOTES

CLIENT

DATE | TIME

PHONE | EMAIL

SERVICE | DURATION

SUPPLIES

NOTES

CLIENT

DATE | TIME

PHONE | EMAIL

SERVICE | DURATION

SUPPLIES

NOTES

CLIENT

DATE | TIME

PHONE | EMAIL

SERVICE | DURATION

SUPPLIES

NOTES

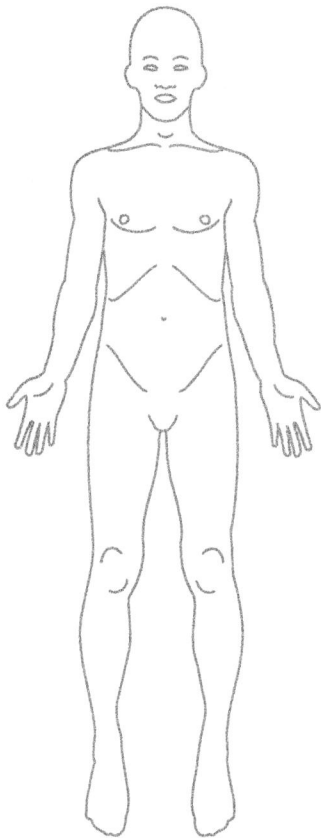

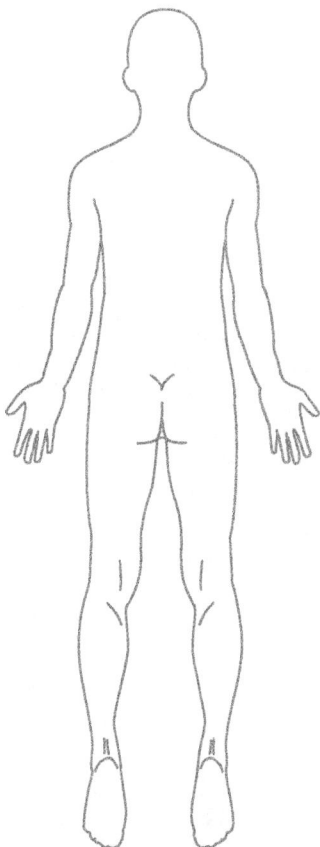

www.ingramcontent.com/pod-product-compliance
Lightning Source LLC
Chambersburg PA
CBHW080601030426
42336CB00019B/3291